Patrícia Queiroz de Lima

Electrochemotherapy in veterinary medicine

Patrícia Queiroz de Lima

Electrochemotherapy in veterinary medicine

ScienciaScripts

Imprint
Any brand names and product names mentioned in this book are subject to trademark, brand or patent protection and are trademarks or registered trademarks of their respective holders. The use of brand names, product names, common names, trade names, product descriptions etc. even without a particular marking in this work is in no way to be construed to mean that such names may be regarded as unrestricted in respect of trademark and brand protection legislation and could thus be used by anyone.

Cover image: www.ingimage.com

This book is a translation from the original published under ISBN 978-620-2-18841-8.

Publisher:
Sciencia Scripts
is a trademark of
Dodo Books Indian Ocean Ltd. and OmniScriptum S.R.L publishing group

120 High Road, East Finchley, London, N2 9ED, United Kingdom
Str. Armeneasca 28/1, office 1, Chisinau MD-2012, Republic of Moldova, Europe
Printed at: see last page
ISBN: 978-620-7-27718-6

Electrochemotherapy in veterinary medicine

Patrícia Queiroz de Lima

Dedication

I dedicate this book to my mum, Teresa, for supporting me in my studies without ever measuring her efforts.

To my husband Danilo, for always being by my side, supporting me in times of joy and difficulty.

Thank you

Firstly, I thank Jehovah God, the creator of everything.

To my sister Kátia for all her support and for contributing to my education.

To my animals, Pingo, Bruce, Vitória, Pérola and Tauriel for all the love, affection and joy shared and passed on to the whole family.

To my dear teacher, master and supervisor Fernanda Paes de Oliveira for all the study and knowledge she passed on.

To the veterinary oncologist Dr Alberto Bajo from the Vet Hospital Firenze - Italy for the images of patients treated with the electrochemotherapy technique.

To all my undergraduate teachers.

The Adamantina University Centre - UNIFAI.

Foreword

The aim of this book is to expand knowledge of this new technique for treating cancer in veterinary medicine.

The book takes an approach that enables the reader to understand the principle of electrochemotherapy, its technique and indications.

The book covers everything from the history of electrochemotherapy to its therapeutic and side effects.

It is not intended to be a book of technical aspects that are difficult to read, so that students of veterinary medicine can better understand and become interested in this new modality of antineoplastic treatment.

It addresses important issues such as the use of electrochemotherapy instead of conventional treatments such as radiotherapy or even intravenous chemotherapy alone.

Years have passed and new studies are emerging, so owners are looking for more sophisticated treatments to prolong their pet's life. Electrochemotherapy is one of these alternatives, saving many lives, with the fewest possible side effects and the shortest treatment time.

Chapter 1: Introduction to electrochemotherapy

1.1 History

In the 1980s, Dr Lluis Mir had the idea of using electroporation to potentiate antineoplastic drugs. Electroporation had previously been widely used in gene transfection experiments, which facilitated the entry of drugs into cells. This led to the creation of a new cancer treatment technique called electrochemotherapy.

Two decades later, in 2006, the technique was standardised for medicine in Europe. Today, this technique is being developed in 83 medical centres around the world, all located in Europe.

In veterinary medicine, the first article on the subject was published in 1997, and today this technique is used in countries such as Italy, England, Slovenia and Brazil.

2.1 Fundamentals of electroporation

Electroporation or electropermeabilisation is a molecular biology technique in which an electric field is applied to cells, increasing the permeability of their membranes and allowing the introduction of drugs (Figure 1).

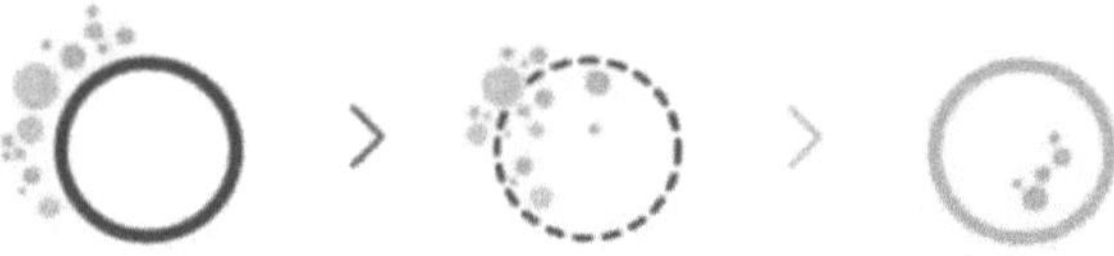

Figure 1. Representation of cell permeability, entry of drug into the cell through the opening of pores. Source: Sciences.

The phenomenon of reversible electrical breaks in the cell membrane was reported by Stampfli in 1958. In the following decade Sale and Hamilton reported non-thermal destruction of microorganisms subjected to high electrical pulses.

In 1972 Newmann and Rosenhech observed an increase in the permeability of vesicles subjected to electrical pulses, and in 1988 an increase in the cytotoxicity of bleomycin was observed in vitro and in vivo with the use of electrical pulses, which came to be called electrochemotherapy.

Electroporation aims to facilitate the entry of non-permeable or poorly permeable substances into the cell membrane. When a cell is subjected to an electric field, there is a difference in transmembrane potential where permeability increases. This phenomenon is called electroporation or electropermeabilisation. The intensity of the induced field will determine the area of electroporation, and the duration and number of pulses will define the size of the pore.

The pores formed by the electric field may be reversible, maintaining the viability of the cell after application. If the amplitude and duration of the electric pulses exceed certain standards that the cell membrane can withstand, the pores become irreversible, causing cell death. Pores form almost immediately after the electric field is applied and close after a few seconds or minutes.

During exposure of the tissue to the electric field there is also a decrease in blood flow, thus allowing more time for the drug to penetrate through the pores formed, which results in a higher intracellular concentration of the drug in the exposed tissue.

Electroporation has been applied in various fields of biochemistry, molecular biology, medicine and oncology. It is used to increase the efficiency of DNA vaccines, to activate immunity against cancer, in electrochemotherapy, in plasmid transfer and cell fusion, transport of molecules and insertion of proteins into the cell membrane.

The application of electroporation promotes the transient formation of a pore by increasing the dipolar moment of hydrophilic lipid heads, allowing macromolecules to migrate through the pores and reach the nucleus, where they can promote genetic transformations. It is a non-invasive method and does not alter the biological structure of the target cell.

There are two types of wave: a square wave, used with a duration of less than 100 ^s, its voltage and duration remain constant; the square wave pulse is used to achieve better control of drug transport. The other wave is the exponential wave, which has an advantage because it maintains or expands the state of high permeability induced by electroporation and promotes electroporetic movement.

2.1.1 Graphical representation of electric

waves

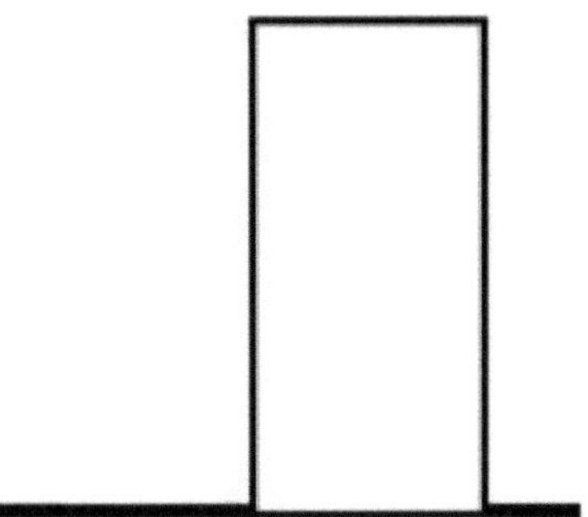

Figure 2. Square wave. Source: www.ibytes.com.br

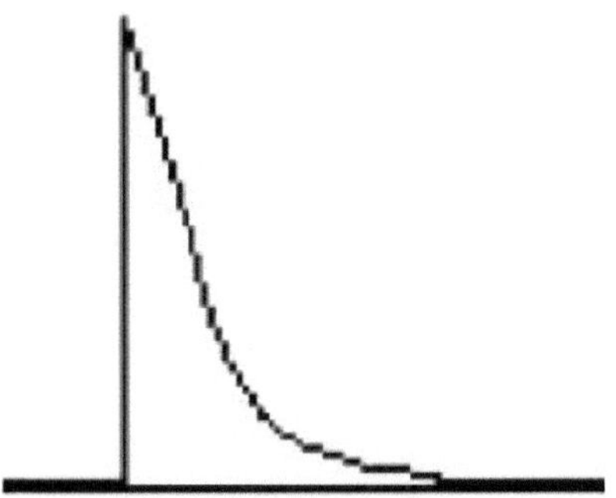

Figure 3. Exponential wave. Source:

www.ibytes.com.br

Chapter 3: Electrochemotherapy procedure

Electrochemotherapy is indicated for the treatment of cutaneous and subcutaneous neoplasms, although there are already reports of the use of this therapeutic method during the transoperative period.

The anaesthetic protocol will depend on the animal's age and physical condition. Once the animal is anaesthetised, the tumour can be better assessed, measured and delimited using a caliper.

The chemotherapeutic agents used in electrochemotherapy are cisplatin and bleomycin.

The chemotherapeutic agent is applied intratumourally or intravenously, then the neoplasm is subjected to electroporation by applying electrical pulses in fractions of a second, the electrode is moved and electroporated until it covers its entire length.

The dose of the drug to be applied intratumourally depends on the volume of the mass, which is calculated using the formula $V = abcn./6,$ where "a", "b" and "c" are the length, width and height of the lesion respectively. The measurements can be taken using a caliper (Figure 4).

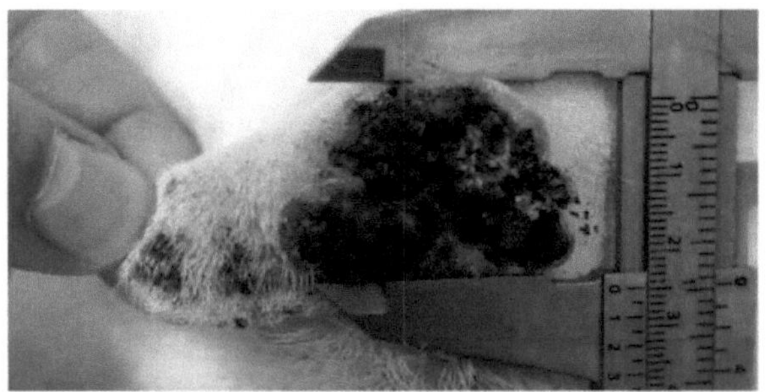

Figure 4: Measurement of tumour size using a caliper.

Source: Dr Alberto Bajo - Italy.

As the aim of electrochemotherapy is to open up the cell membrane for the local action of the chemotherapeutic drug, cell death is caused by the cytotoxic agent and not by electricity, as it only increases cell permeability to the drug chosen for treatment.

3.1 Bleomycin

Bleomycin was first discovered in 1966, when Japanese scientist Hamao Umezawa discovered anti-cancer activity while screening *Streptomyces Verticillus* culture filtrates.

Umezawa published his discovery in 1966, and the drug was launched in Japan by Nippon Kayaku in 1969.

In the USA, bleomycin was approved for marketing in July 1973, initially by the Bristol-Myers Squibb precursor, Bristol Laboratories, under the brand name Blenoxane.

Bleomycin acts by binding to DNA and breaking the DNA strand.

It acts mainly in the G2 and M phases of the cell cycle.

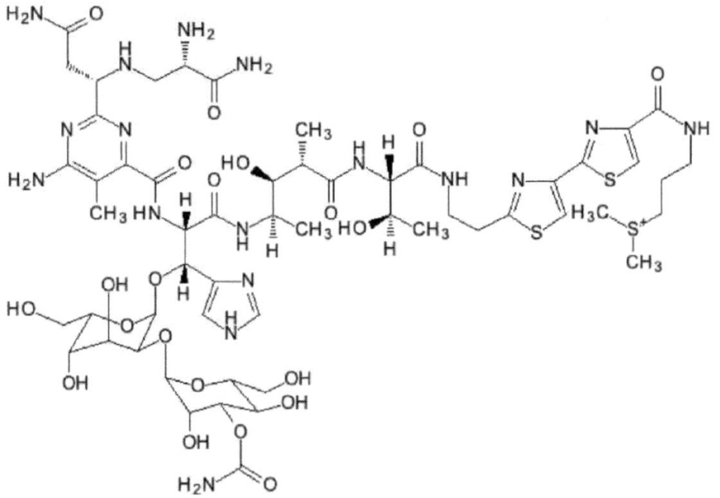

Figure 5 - Representation of the chemical formula of the drug bleomycin. Source: Wikipedia

Bleomycin can be administered intravenously or intratumourally.

The dose and intervals between injections depend on the indication, method

of administration, age and physical condition of the patient. For intravenous

administration, the required dose should be dissolved in 5 to 1000ml of 0.9%

sodium chloride and injected slowly. Bleomycin for intratumoural use

should be dissolved in 0.9% sodium chloride in concentrations of 1 to 3x,

103 IU/ml of solution.

In veterinary medicine, bleomycin is indicated for the treatment of splenic neoplasms, lymphomas, carcinomas and mastocytomas. Blenoxam is presented for use in animals in ampoule vials containing 15 units. The dose for cats is 0.3 to 0.5U/kg weekly IM, SC, IV. The dose for dogs is $10U/m^2$ IV or SC, once a day for 3 to 4 days and then weekly up to a maximum dose of 125 to 200mg/m2.

The main route of excretion of bleomycin is via the kidney, with 60 to 70 per cent of an administered dose recovered in the urine as active bleomycin. Animals with renal deficiencies can significantly prolong excretion.

The side effects of intravenous and intramuscular administration of bleomycin include: anorexia, vomiting, hair loss, pulmonary toxicity is the most serious side effect, occurring in 10% of patients treated with this drug, approximately 1% can suffer non-specific pneumonitis induced by bleomycin, evolution to pulmonary fibrosis and death can occur, but pulmonary toxicity has a higher incidence in elderly patients. The first symptom associated with pulmonary toxicity is dyspnoea.

2.2 Cisplatin

Cisplatin was synthesised in 1844 by Michel Peyrone. In 1893 its structure was elucidated by Alfred Werner and in 1960 it was rediscovered through experiments carried out in the laboratories of Michigan State University by Bernett Rosenberg, who was studying the effect of an electric current on the bacterial growth of *Escherichia Coli.*

It was concluded that the mitosis of bacteria was inhibited not by electrical phenomena, but by a chemical agent, cisplatin. In 1970, the effects of cisplatin were tested and proven in artificially implanted sarcomas in rats, followed by toxicity tests carried out on dogs and monkeys.

In 1972 the National Cancer Institute introduced it into clinical trials and in 1978 it was approved for clinical use by the FDA (Food and Drug Administration).

Cisplatin's antitumour activity is attributed to DNA binding, inducing structural changes. Its cytotoxic effect is caused by inhibition of transcription and replication, thus inducing apoptosis.

Protein and RNA synthesis are also affected, but to a lesser extent. Cisplatin was recognised as a cancer treatment drug in 1973.

Cisplatin should be used with caution as it is highly nephrotoxic and cannot be administered IV in cats.

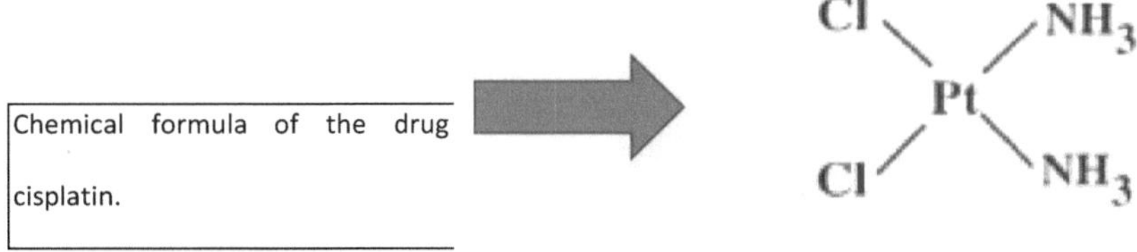

Figure 6 - Representation of the chemical formula of the drug cisplatin. Source: Staff.

3.3 Preventive measures for preparing drugs

Professionals must take preventive measures when handling chemotherapy drugs, due to the risks of exposure they present. The drug should be prepared in an environment free of air flow, preferably using a laminar flow cabinet or biological safety cabinet (Figure 7), wearing a pair of latex gloves, long-sleeved aprons, a cap, a mask and goggles.

Handling should be done as far away from the face as possible, dispose of materials immediately after use.

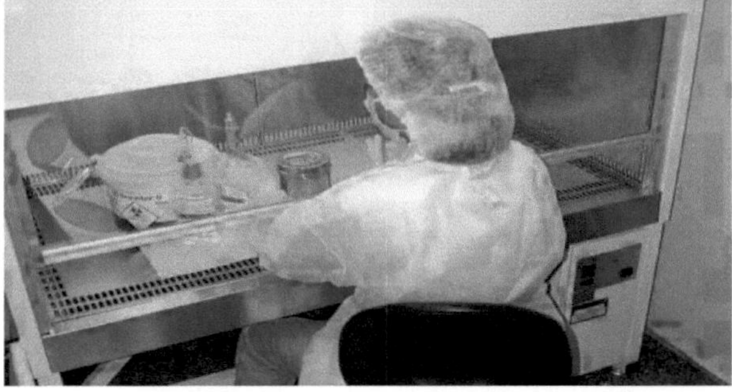

Figure 7. Biological safety cabinet, designed to prevent direct contact, provides protection for the professional and the external environment. Source: www.biosseguranca.com.br

3.4 Electroporator

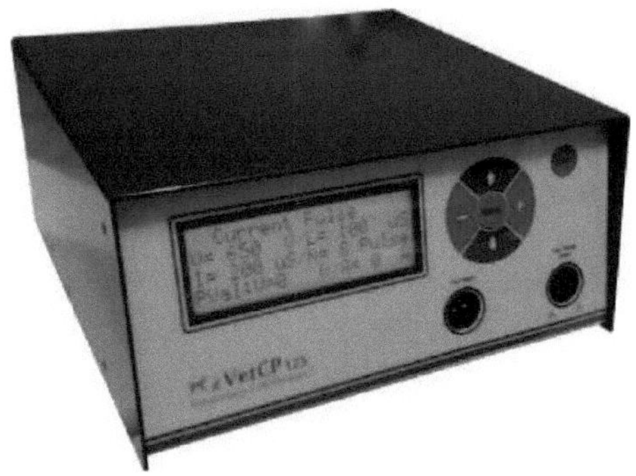

Figure 8. Vet CP125 electroporator. Source: Vet Câncer - Brazil.

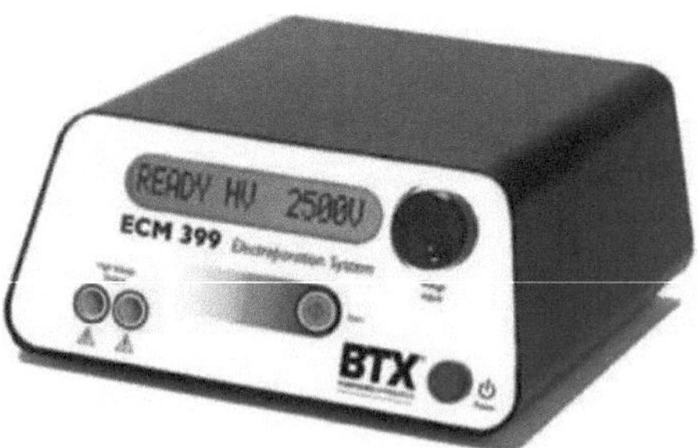

Figure 9. BTX ECM399 electroporator. Source: www.analiticaweb.com.br

For electrochemotherapy, the electric currents generated by the electroporator are high voltage, and the results are best when this voltage ranges from 800 to 1500 volts. The electrical pulses have to be of microsecond duration ranging from 20 to 1000^s at a frequency of 1 Hertz with a frequency of 8 pulses.

The electric current is applied using electrodes with a flat surface or in the form of equidistant needles (Figures 10 and 11), so electrochemotherapy is used in areas affected by neoplasms, but with very limited surgical margins.

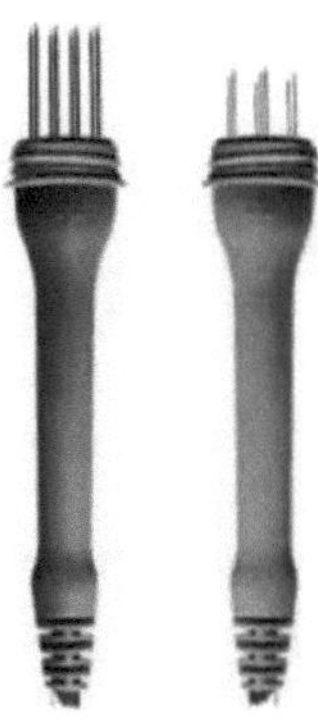

Figure 10. Electrodes on equidistant needles. Source: www.sciencedirect.com

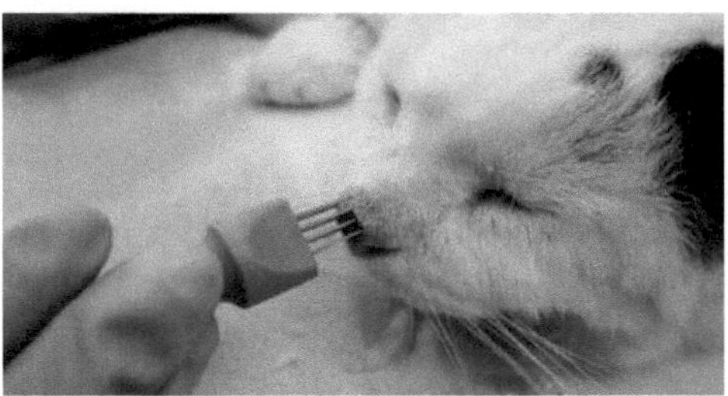

Figure 11. Electrodes on a needle during an electrochemotherapy session. Source: Dr Alberto

Bajo - Italy.

Electrochemotherapy has been shown to be effective in the treatment of cutaneous and subcutaneous neoplasms, whether benign or malignant. This chapter will look at the main neoplasms indicated for electrochemotherapy.

4.1 Squamous cell carcinoma

Squamous cell carcinoma, also known as squamous cell carcinoma, is very common in tropical countries. This neoplasm usually occurs due to excessive exposure to ultraviolet radiation. It is a malignant neoplasm of the keratinocytes, slow-growing and not necessarily metastatic, and its occurrence is very common in light-coated animals.

The main reason for the appearance of this neoplasm is chronic exposure to ultraviolet rays, hairlessness and lack of pigmentation. They are common neoplasms in all species and can occur in young animals, but the incidence increases with age.

Solar dermatosis is the first sign of the development of the disease, and erythema, oedema and peeling of the skin are still observed, followed by the formation of crusts and ulceration. As the neoplasm progresses, the tumour becomes firmer, and as a result the ulcers increase, which can lead to secondary bacterial contamination, resulting in purulent exudate on the tumour surface.

Squamous cell carcinoma in cats has the highest incidence, with lesions usually occurring in the nasal planum (Figure 12), eyelids and ears (Figure 13).

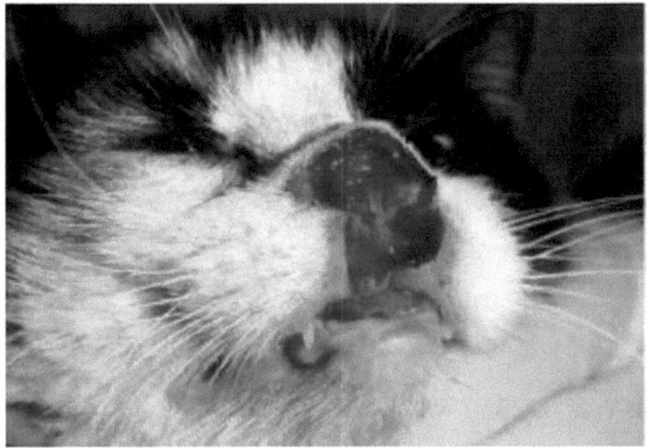

Figure 12. Squamous cell carcinoma in the nasal plane of a cat. Source: UFP - Brazil.

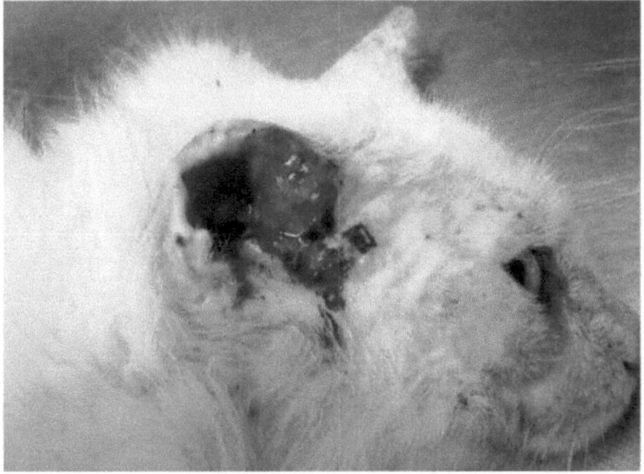

Figure 13. Squamous cell carcinoma in the ear of a cat.

Source: www.centromedicoveterinario.com.br

In the early stages, surgery, cryotherapy, radiotherapy or chemotherapy are treatment options. In the advanced stages, surgery can affect the animal's aesthetics, while radiotherapy can cause conjunctivitis, ulcerative keratitis and dry keratoconjunctivitis.

Electrochemotherapy has been shown to be effective in treating squamous cell carcinoma in cats (Figures 14, 15, 16 and 17).

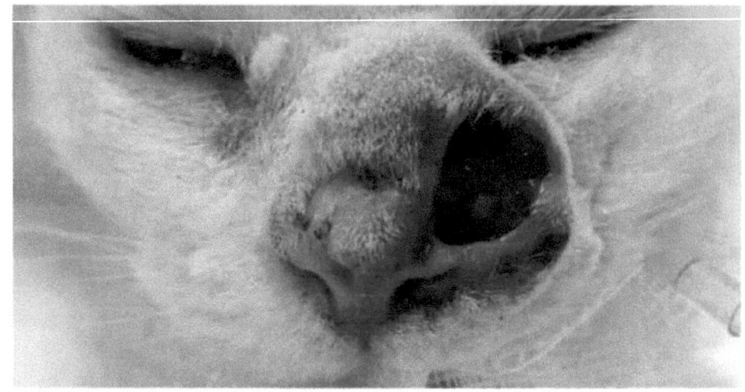

Figura 14.   Squamous cell carcinoma in a cat before starting treatment with electrochemotherapy. Source: Dr Alberto Bajo - Italy.

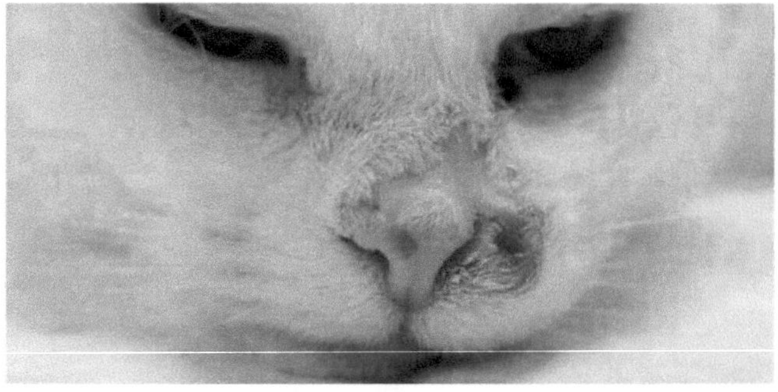

Figura 15.   Squamous cell carcinoma in a cat after treatment with electrochemotherapy. Source: Dr Alberto Bajo - Italy.

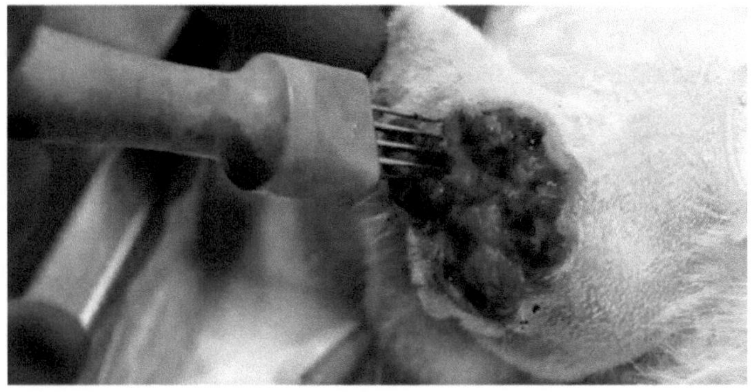

Figura 16.   Squamous cell carcinoma in a cat's ear during the first session of

electrochemotherapy. Source: Dr Alberto Bajo - Italy

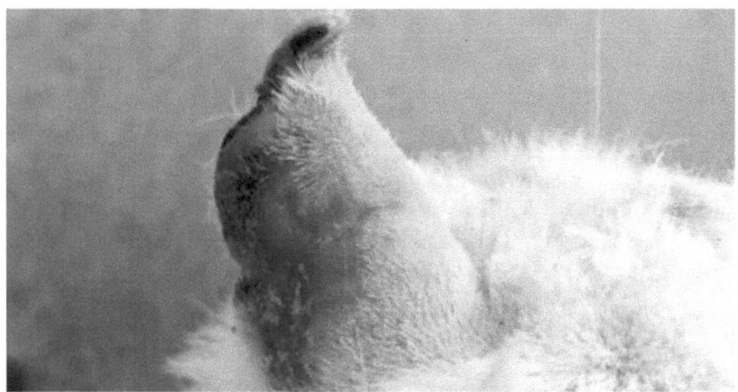

Figura 17.   Squamous cell carcinoma in a cat's ear after a few sessions of

electrochemotherapy. Source: Dr Alberto Bajo - Italy.

4.2 Perianal neoplasms

The perianal gland is a sebaceous gland located next to the anus, on the side, which has the function of lubricating faeces. These glands can undergo changes, becoming neoplasms consisting of adenomas and adenocarcinomas.

4.2.1 Perianal adenoma

The development of adenomas and adenocarcinomas is influenced by gonadal hormones, basically testosterone. Due to the influence of this hormone, perianal tumours are common in male dogs and rare in cats.

Perianal adenomas account for 80% of neoplasms and are the third most common in entire animals, with the highest incidence occurring in geriatric dogs (between 8 and 12 years old). Adenomas can also affect females due to the influence of oestrogen.

Macroscopically, this neoplasm is seen as solitary or multiple nodules or masses, which can vary in size and may be ulcerated (Figure 18).

Perianal adenomas are benign neoplasms, which facilitates treatment and the animal's outlook on life. Surgical removal, radiotherapy and conventional chemotherapy have proven to be very effective, but electrochemotherapy has shown greater efficacy with shorter treatment times and fewer side effects (Figure 19).

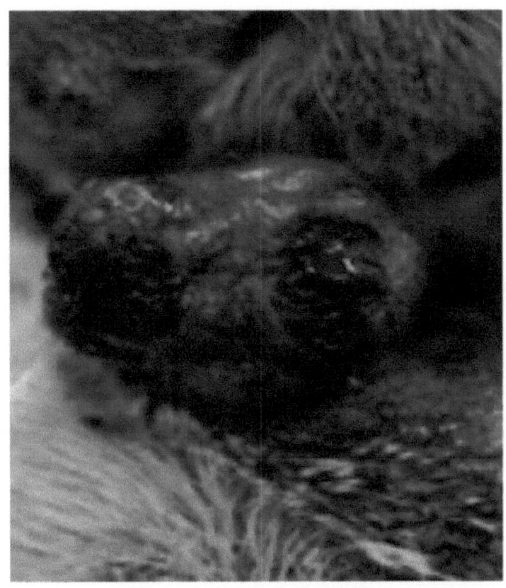

Figure 18. Perianal adenoma before treatment with electrochemotherapy.

Source: Dr Alberto Bajo - Italy.

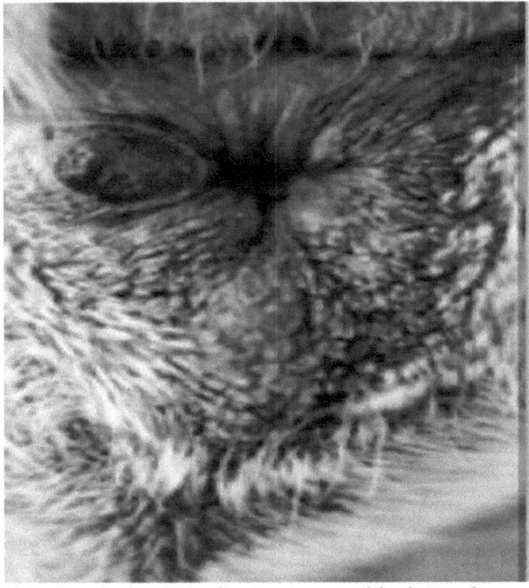

Figure 19. Perianal adenoma after treatment with electrochemotherapy.

Source: Dr Alberto Bajo - Italy.

4.2.2 Perianal adenocarcinoma

Adenocarcinoma is a malignant neoplasm of the perianal glands of animals, mainly elderly male dogs. This neoplasm occurs less frequently than perianal adenoma.

This neoplasm is characterised by being regionally invasive and can proliferate in the abdominal lymph nodes and produce hepatic, splenic, renal and pulmonary metastases. This neoplasm affects whole and sterilised males and there is no hormonal influence on this type of neoplasm.

Surgical removal is the treatment of choice for this neoplasm, but surgical excisions in this region can cause complications such as infection and suture dehiscence, damage to the anal sphincter, fibrosis and anal stenosis. Chemotherapy and radiotherapy have not shown encouraging results for this type of tumour. The use of electrochemotherapy has been shown to be effective as it does not cause anatomical or functional alterations to the region and does not cause pharmacological toxicity.

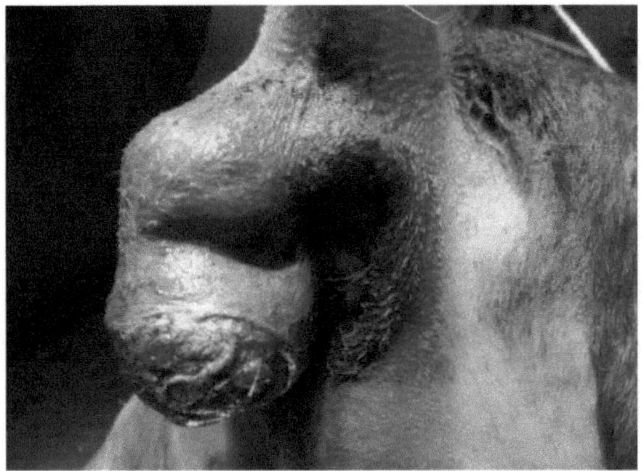

Figure 20. Perianal adenocarcinoma in a dog. Source: Campinas Veterinary Medical Centre.

4.3 Melanoma

Melanoma is a neoplasm that originates in melanocytes. It is one of the types of cancer with the worst prognosis and a high incidence of metastases. It originates through the transformation of melanocytes (cells responsible for producing melanin, which blocks ultraviolet rays).

The formation of melanoma involves several stages, from small spots on the skin, through abnormal cell proliferation to the formation of an invasive and metastatic tumour. Melanoma can occur in the mouth, head, scrotum, limbs, intraocular (Figure 21), with no distinction between age or gender.

Dog breeds such as the Boxer, Airedale, Chihuahua, Golden Retriever, Labrador Retriever, Doberman, Pinscher and Chow Chow have a higher risk of developing this type of neoplasm.

In cats, it commonly occurs on the eyelids, intraoculars, ears, lips, muzzle, neck and limbs, and can affect cats of any age and sex.

The treatment of choice is surgical removal, but it is common for the disease to reappear. Radiotherapy associated with surgical removal has shown good results. Chemotherapy helps control the disease, but does not cure it alone. The drugs used for this type of neoplasm are carboplatin, cisplatin, doxorubicin and non-steroidal anti-inflammatory drugs.

Immunotherapy has demonstrated its progress in veterinary medicine against cancer, as a new product has been approved for use called the Oncept® vaccine from Merial to treat stage 2 and 3 oral melanoma in dogs. This vaccine stimulates the production of the enzyme tyrosinase, which induces the animal's immune system to identify the neoplastic melanoma cells and destroy them. This vaccine has shown satisfactory results and given animals with this neoplasm a longer survival time.

Electrochemotherapy against melanoma has the capacity to regress the tumour by up to 90%, increasing the animal's survival rate to more than 360 days. However, its use is limited and its results are promising in superficial cutaneous melanoma.

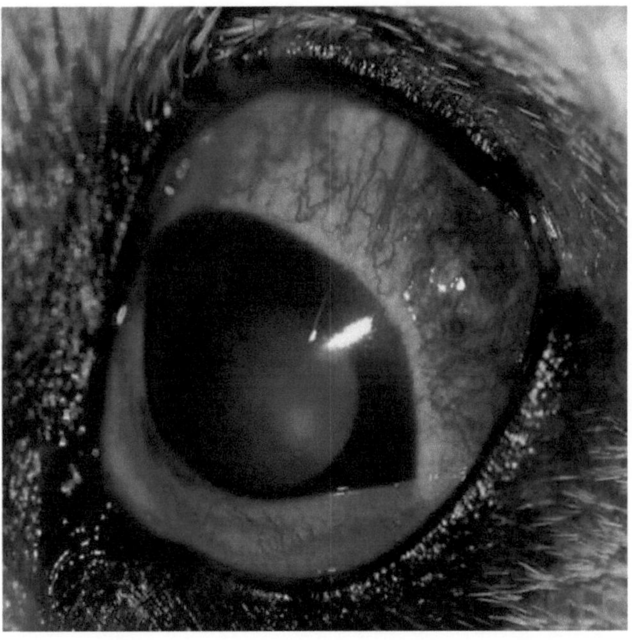

Figure 21. Intraocular melanoma in a labrador breed dog. Source: IVO, Institute of Veterinary Ophthalmology - Spain

4.4 Melanocytomas

Melanocytomas originate from melanocytes and melanoblasts. Melanocytes are cells derived from melanoblasts that have migrated to the epidermis, dermis, mucous membranes and choroid during embryogenesis. They are found in the skin, in the basal layer of the epidermis, dispersed among the basal keratinocytes.

This neoplasm, also known as cutaneous melanoma, has no known or proven metastatic potential, but most are benign and do not cause metastases. The lesion occurs on the hind limbs and head of animals, is a common neoplasm in elderly animals and is more common in males. The lesion is dark in colour with pigment or can be light in colour, with small lesions occurring.

Treatment is the same as for melanoma, but there is no recurrence rate and treatment takes less time when electrochemotherapy is used as a curative method.

1.5 Mastocytomas

Mastocytoma is a malignant neoplasm caused by the differentiation of mast cells (cells that act in the immune system of the skin and mucous membranes, releasing histamine and heparin granules). On macroscopy, mastocytomas can be lobulated, firm, soft, ulcerated or not. It is a highly metastatic neoplasm and can affect the lymph nodes, spleen, liver and bone marrow. Breeds such as the Boxer, Boston Terrier, Beagle, Bulldog, Labrador, Golden Retriever, Pit Bull, Sharpei and dogs without a defined breed are predisposed to this neoplastic formation. There is no sexual predisposition, and as far as age is concerned, young dogs are affected, but elderly dogs aged between 7 and 9 years have the highest incidence.

The lesions can be nodules, masses or erythematous, poorly delimited, firm, ulcerated, adherent and infiltrative plaques (Figure 22). When found in the subcutaneous tissue, they can be mistaken for lipomas due to their soft, floating appearance.

Treatment is based on surgical excision, chemotherapy, radiotherapy and electrochemotherapy. The response to chemotherapy treatment has been unsatisfactory in terms of tumour regression. The use of electrochemotherapy has shown satisfactory results due to its non-invasive and painless therapeutic mode (Figure 23).

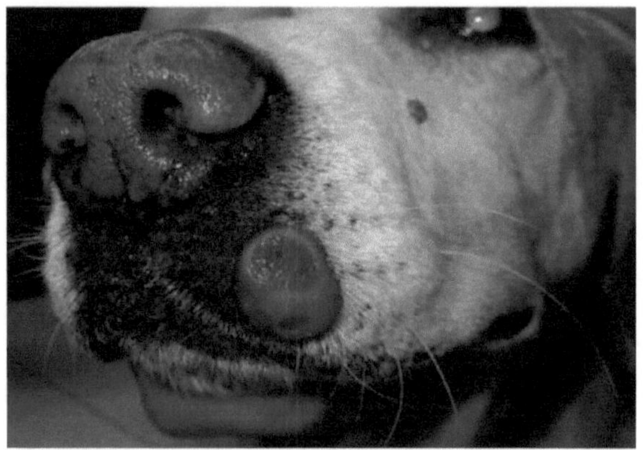

Figure 22. Mastocytoma in a dog. Source:

www.oncologiaveterinaria.it

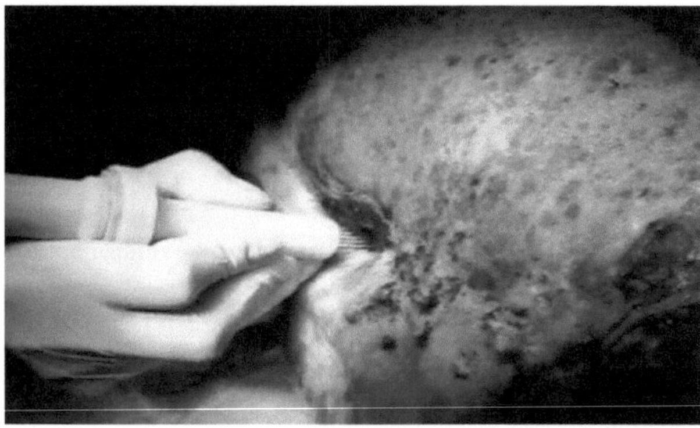

Figure 23. Electrochemotherapy in cutaneous mastocytoma in a dog. Source: Dr Carlos

Brunner - Brazil.

1.6 Transmissible Venereal Tumour (TVT)

Also known as Sticker's tumour, the transmissible venereal tumour is a malignant neoplasm transmitted between dogs through direct contact, mainly through coitus, and has low metastatic potential. On macroscopy, this neoplasm is an ulcerated mass with a cauliflower-like appearance that affects the genitals as well as the oral cavity, auditory pavilion, spleen, liver, kidney, snout, lung, skin, anal region, pharynx, brain, ovaries and foreskin, albeit less frequently. They can be solitary or multiple, friable, haemorrhagic and/or necrotic (Figures 24 and 25).

There is no racial or sexual predisposition for the disease to develop, most of those affected are sexually active animals. In females, it usually develops during oestrus when the vulvar blood supply is high, favouring the implantation of neoplastic cells.

Surgical excision is effective in some animals, but recurrence is a

problem.

frequent. The treatment of choice for this type of neoplasm is the

administration of the chemotherapy drug Vincristine, which has shown

satisfactory results in a short period of time, causes few side effects and the

cure rate is approximately 100%. However, electrochemotherapy has proved

successful in the treatment of TVT. In just one session, the neoplasm shrinks

by 70 to 100 per cent and is cured without recurrence.

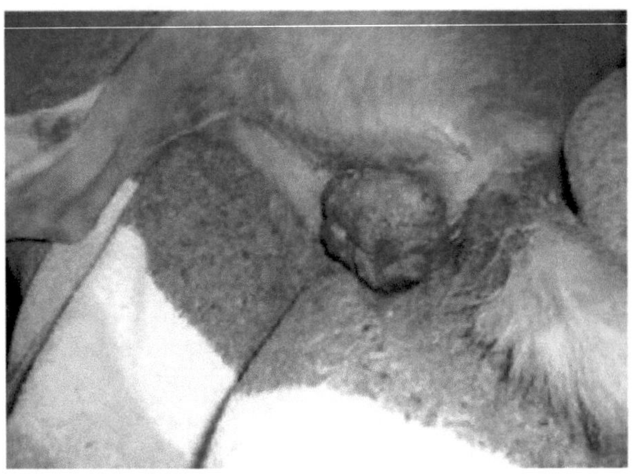

Figure 24. Vulvar DVT in a female dog. Source: Petcare - Brazil.

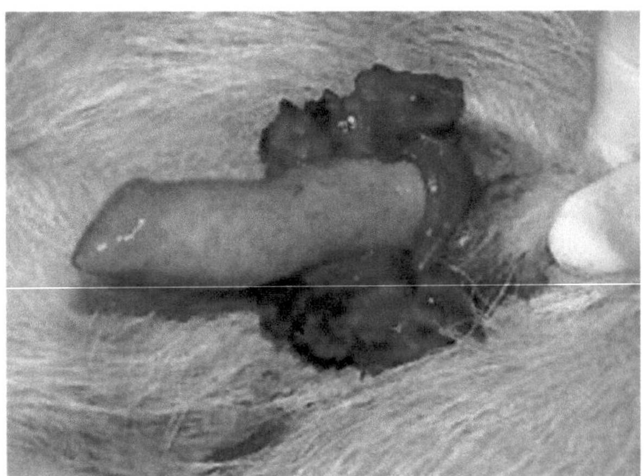

Figure 25. Penile DVT in a dog. Source: www.webanimal.com.br

1.7 Cutaneous haemangiosarcoma

It is a highly malignant endothelial cell neoplasm, commonly found in the spleen, liver, heart and skin. It can originate from any highly vascularised organ or tissue, and its main target for metastasis is the lungs. Animals with little pigment in their skin and prolonged exposure to ultraviolet rays tend to develop this type of neoplasm. On macroscopy, cutaneous haemangiosarcoma has a discreet, firm, raised shape, dark to purple haemorrhagic subcutaneous nodules or masses (Figure 26), and there are usually no ulcerations. When the muscles are invaded, swelling and oedema may occur.

The treatment of choice is surgical excision associated with chemotherapy, but the toxicity of the drug used, such as doxorubicin, can worsen the animal's condition. Palliative radiotherapy is rarely used, but it has been shown to reduce the size of the tumour, but does not increase the animal's survival. Electrochemotherapy has been shown to have a high curative potential, increasing the animal's life expectancy in cutaneous haemangiosarcoma without signs of metastasis.

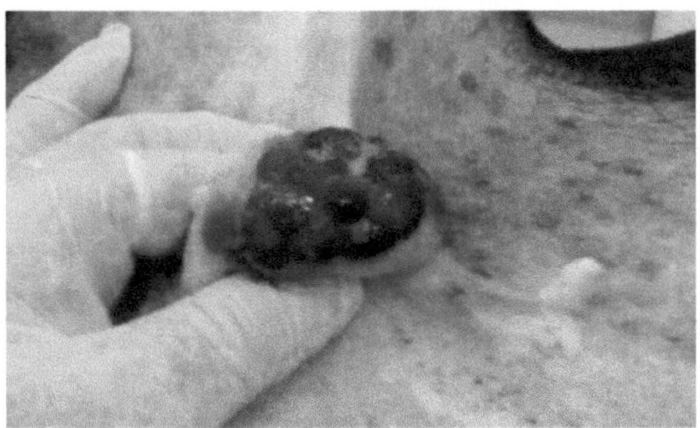

Figure 26. Cutaneous haemangiosarcoma in a Pitbull dog. Source:

www.carlosmorales.wordpress.com

5.1 Equine sarcoid

Equine sarcoid is the most common cutaneous neoplasm in horses, usually affecting animals under 4 years of age, with no predilection for breed, sex or coat. The neoplastic lesions occur in the periocular region (Figure 27), cervical region, limbs and ventral region of the animal's body. On macroscopy, the lesions are multiple and can appear suddenly and disappear in the same way. This neoplasm does not metastasise but has a high recurrence rate.

Equine sarcoid is a neoplasm of fibrous tissue with a fibroblastic origin and a low rate of metastasis. Although there is no breed predilection, horses of the Appaloosa, Purebred Arabian, Purebred English, Quarter Horse and Criollo breeds are the most affected.

Surgical excision has not shown good results due to the high rate of recurrence of equine sarcoid, but electrochemotherapy (Figure 28) has shown satisfactory results, with no recurrence with this therapeutic method. As a result, many horses are cured of this type of neoplasm in a short period of time without the need for surgical intervention, which often ends up interfering with the animal's aesthetics.

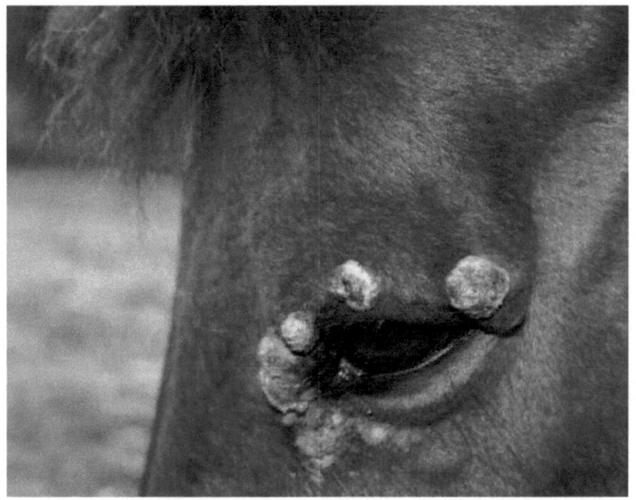

Figure 27. Periocular equine sarcoid. Source:www.classequine.com

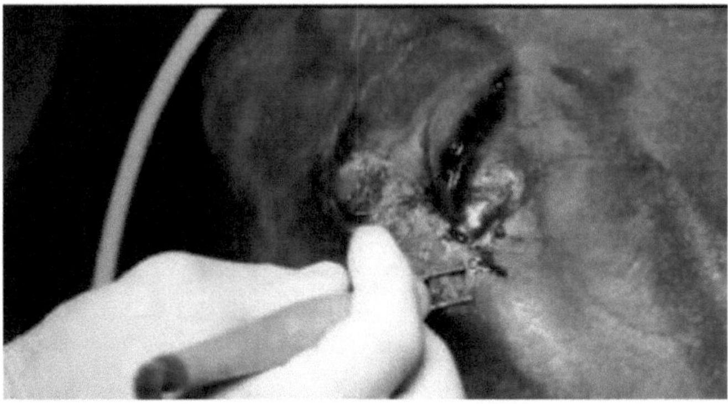

Figure 28. Electrochemotherapy procedure on periocular sarcoid. Source: Clinique

Equine de Bordeaux - France.

Electrochemotherapy has no significant side effects. Involuntary muscle contractions at the site of application of the electrical pulses cease at the end of the procedure, after the sessions, most patients show normal behaviour, inflammatory reactions may be present with slight erythema in the adjacent normal tissue, superficial crust formation may be observed in the first few days after application, in larger tumours ulcerations may occur in the neoplastic nodule, both lesions should disappear within five days of treatment.

Chapter 7 Final considerations

Currently, electrochemotherapy has been shown to be very effective in various types of neoplasms. Compared to radiotherapy, conventional chemotherapy and surgery, it has had a greater advantage due to the fact that it has no significant side effects. However, it has low success rates in neoplasms with bone involvement and lacks accessibility in very large tumours that make it impossible to electroporate their entire volume.

Therefore, this new therapeutic method has increased the quality and lifespan of animals with malignant neoplasms, as relapses after treatment are rarely reported, demonstrating the high efficacy of this technique.

References
AMINKOV, B.; MANOV, V. **Electrochemotherapy**: a novel method od treatment of malignant tumours in the dog. Bulg Vet Med, 2004.

DALECK, C.R.; DE NARDI, A.B. **Oncology in dogs and cats**. Rio de Janeiro: Roca, 2016.

DALECK, C.R.; DE NARDI, A.B.; RODASKI, S. **Oncology in dogs and cats**. 1. ed. São Paulo: Roca, 2009.

GEHL, J. **Electroporation:** theory and methods, perspective for drug delivery, gene therapy and research. **Acta physiologica Scandinavica**, 2003.

GOTHELF, A.; MIR, L, M.; GEHL, J. **Electrochemotherapy:** results of cancer treatment using enhanced delivery of bleomycin by electroporation. **Cancer treatment reviwe**, v.29, n.5, p.371-387, 2003.

JUNQUEIRA, L.C.; CARNEIRO, J. **Basic histology.** 10.ed. Rio de Janeiro: Guanabara Koogan, 2004.

LAUS, J.L. **Clinical and surgical ophthalmology in dogs and cats**. São Paulo: Roca, 2009. ch.5, p. 97-110.

MCGAVIN, M.D.; ZACHARY, J.F. **Basis of veterinary pathology**. 4.ed. Rio de Janeiro: Elsevier, 2009. chap.20.

MIR, L, M. Bases and rationale of electrochemotherapy, **European Journal**

of Cancer Supplements, v.4, p.38-44, 2006.

PAGE, R.L.; THRALL, D.C. Soft tissue sarcomas and haemangiosarcomas. In: ETTINGER, S.J.; FELDMAN, E.C. **Treatise on veterinary internal medicine**. Rio de Janeiro: Guanabara Koogan, 2004. p.561-566p.

RODARSKI, S.; DE NARDI, A.B. **Antineoplastic chemotherapy in dogs and cats.** 3.ed. São Paulo: Medvet, 2008.

ROGERS, K.S. Chemotherapy of neoplastic diseases. In: ADAMS, H.R. **Farmacologia e terapêutica em veterinária**. Rio de Janeiro: Guanabara Koogan, 2003. 900p.

SANTOS, J. A. **General pathology of domestic animals**. 3.ed. Rio de Janeiro: Guanabara, 1998. p.314-315.

SERSA, G.; CEMAZAR, M.; SNOJ, M. Electrochemotherapy of tumours. **Radiology and Oncology**, 2006.

SILVEIRA, L. M. G.; BRUNNER, C.H.M. Use of electrochemotherapy in neoplasms of epithelial or mesenchymal origin located on the skin or mucous membranes of dogs. **Brazilian Journal of Veterinary Research and Animal Science**, v.47, n.1, p.55-66, 2010.

SPUGNINI, E.P.; BALDI, A. Electrochemotherapy in veterinary oncology: **From rescue to first live therapy**, 2014.

TELLÓ, M. et al. **The use of electric current in cancer treatment**. 3.ed. Porto Alegre: EDIPUCRS, 2004. p.77-96.

UGEN, K.E.; HELLER, R. Electroporation as a method for the efficient in vivo deliveryof therapeutic genes. **DNA and Cell Biology**, 2003.

Table of contents

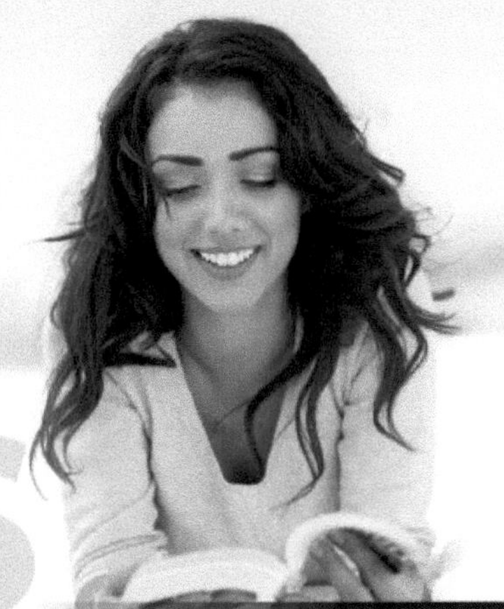

yes
I want morebooks!

Buy your books fast and straightforward online - at one of world's fastest growing online book stores! Environmentally sound due to Print-on-Demand technologies.

Buy your books online at
www.morebooks.shop

Kaufen Sie Ihre Bücher schnell und unkompliziert online – auf einer der am schnellsten wachsenden Buchhandelsplattformen weltweit! Dank Print-On-Demand umwelt- und ressourcenschonend produziert.

Bücher schneller online kaufen
www.morebooks.shop

info@omniscriptum.com
www.omniscriptum.com

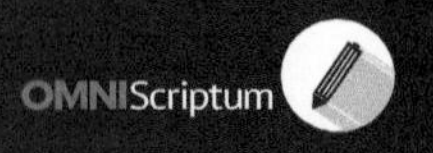

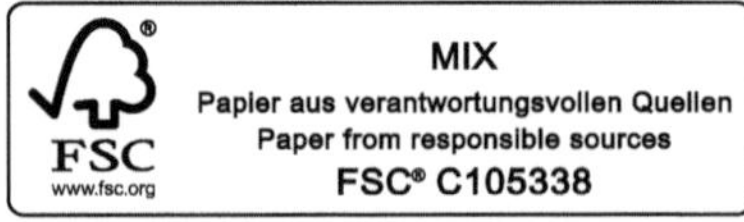

Printed by Books on Demand GmbH, Norderstedt / Germany